DIVERTICULITIS

Diet

COOKBOOK

Discover Healthy, Delicious, And Easy Recipes for People Living with Diverticulitis

JOAN R. COTTRELL

i

SCAN ME FOR MORE
COOKBOOKS

Table of Contents

Include lots of high-fiber foods in your diet, such as fruits, vegetables, whole grains, and legumes. These meals support regular bowel motions and reduce constipation, which can worsen diverticulitis.

Introduction

Sarah was caught up in a health condition known as Diverticulitis. It started with persistent abdominal pain, bloating, and inconsistent bowel motions. Frustration and suffering became constant companions, threatening to put a pall over her daily existence. Little did she know that a journey toward a healthy lifestyle was about to begin in her life.

Her turning point started when she discovered a treasure trove of nutritious recipes for managing and controlling Diverticulitis. Intrigued and eager, she resolved to embark on a gastronomic excursion that would not only satisfy her palate but also alleviate her ailments. The recipes were carefully created to contain ingredients that are gentle on the digestive system while yet providing necessary nutrients.

One important aspect of her newfound culinary adventure was the emphasis on high-fiber foods. Sarah discovered that fiber could help her manage Diverticulitis. Whole grains, fruits, and vegetables were staples in her diet, replacing processed and low-fiber foods. These small changes made a significant difference since fiber improved her bowel movements and general digestive health.

Sarah experimented with using herbs to add flavor to her food. This resulted in a cornucopia of health benefits. As she began to explore the kitchen, she found the benefits of lean protein. Grilled chicken, fish, and tofu were her protein-rich companions, aiding in the healing process while easing her digestive system.

However, the route to managing Diverticulitis went beyond diet and included adopting a healthy lifestyle. Regular exercise became an unavoidable part of Sarah's regimen. Simple exercises like brisk walking, yoga, and mild strength training not only helped her maintain a healthy weight but also enhanced her entire well-being.

Sarah's experience demonstrates the transformational potential of mindful eating and a balanced lifestyle. By introducing Diverticulitis-friendly dishes into her daily routine and adopting better behaviors, she did not only manage but thrived even with Diverticulitis. Her story serves as an encouragement to others facing similar health issues.

If you, too, want to live a more vibrant life, the solution is right in front of you. Within the pages of the "Diverticulitis Diet Cookbook: Discover Healthy, Delicious, and Easy Recipes for People Living with Diverticulitis," you will discover the same secrets that changed Sarah's and many others' lives.

Let this book be your guide to a future filled with health, flavor, and the unlimited delight of a Diverticulitis diet journey. Your story of wellness and rebirth will be written too; let it start here.

Diverticulitis Diet Tips

I. GENERAL TIPS:

1. **Focus On Fiber Intake**: Eat 25-35 grams of fiber each day from fruits, vegetables, whole grains, and legumes. To prevent gas and bloating, gradually increase your consumption of fiber.

2. **Drink Water**: Drink plenty of water throughout the day to keep your stool soft and avoid constipation. Aim for 8 to 10 glasses every day.

3. **Listen To Your Body**: Pay close attention to your body. Avoid foods that cause symptoms such as bloating, discomfort, and diarrhea.

4. **Cook At Home**: Cooking at home gives you control over the ingredients and portion levels.

5. **Read Product Labels**: Always Check food labels for fiber and hidden sugars.

6. **Change Your Eating Pattern**: Eat smaller and more frequent meals, this can aid digestion and reduce bloating.

7. **Manage Stress**: Stress can worsen stomach problems. Practice calming techniques like yoga or meditation.

II. DURING FLARE-UPS:

1. **Clear liquids**: For a few days, rest your digestive system by drinking clear liquids such as broth, water, and herbal teas.

2. **Low-Fiber Foods:** Low-fiber foods include white bread, rice, pasta, eggs, and lean protein, which should be introduced gradually.

3. **Resist Irritants:** Stay away from spicy meals, coffee, alcohol, and fizzy beverages.

III. LONG-TERM MANAGEMENT:

Maintain A High-Fiber Diet: Continue to eat fiber-rich meals to avoid future flare-ups.

Variety Is Vital: Include a variety of fruits, veggies, and whole grains in your diet to acquire diverse nutrients and fiber.

Limit Your Intake of Processed Foods: Limit your intake of processed foods, which are generally poor in fiber and heavy in unhealthy fats and sugars.

Regular Exercise: Physical activity can help regulate digestion and reduce stress.

Follow-Up Appointments: Make regular visits to your doctor to assess your progress and manage your Diverticulitis.

Part I: Diet to prevent flare-ups

This is the first phase of the three phases of dealing with Diverticulitis. Foods to include in the initial phase of a Diverticulitis flare-up include:

a) Broth

b) Fruit juices without pulp, such as apple juice

c) Gelatin and ice chips.

d) Ice pops with no fruit or pulp

e) Cream-free tea or coffee

f) Plain water

The liquid diet should only be followed for a few days before moving on to the next phase.

Choose skinless chicken, fish, tofu, and beans. These contain important nutrients without excessive fat, which might aggravate symptoms.

Breakfast Recipes

Tropical Sunrise

Ingredients:

- 1 cup frozen pineapple chunks
- 1/2 cup of frozen mango chunks
- 1/4 cup peeled, diced papaya (or 1/4 cup frozen papaya chunks)
- One banana, peeled and cut
- 1/2 cup unsweetened plain yogurt (Greek yogurt is advised for more protein)
- 1/4 cup unsweetened plant-based milk (almond, coconut, or oat milk are excellent choices)
- Add 1/4 cup water or ice cubes as needed
- 1/2 teaspoon of ground ginger
- 1/4 teaspoon of turmeric powder

Directions:

1. Gather all the ingredients.
2. Blend all of the ingredients until smooth. Add more water or ice cubes as needed to achieve the desired consistency.
3. Pour into a glass and drink immediately!

Green Boost

Prep time: 10 minutes.
Total time: 10 minutes.
Servings:2

Ingredients:

- 2 cups fresh spinach (or frozen)
- 1 tiny banana
- 1 small green apple
- 1 orange.
- 1 tbsp chia seeds
- 1 1/2 cups oat milk (or almond milk)

Directions:

1. To prepare, peel and cut the banana into chunks.
2. Peel the orange by hand or with a knife, then cut it into pieces.
3. Wash the apple and remove the core (keeping the peel on).
4. Put all of the ingredients in a blender.
5. Blend the ingredients in a high-speed blender for 1-2 minutes until they are smooth and creamy.
6. If the smoothie is too thick for your taste, add more oat milk (or almond milk).
7. Pour into a cup, bottle, or Mason jar.
8. Enjoy immediately, or refrigerate for up to 24 hours.

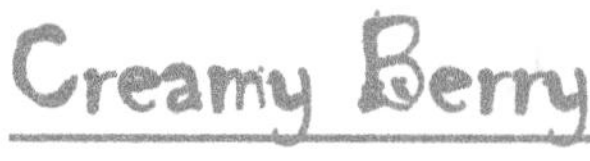

Creamy Berry

Prep time: 10 minutes.
Cook time: 10 minutes.
Total:20minutes
Servings:8

Ingredients:

- 1 cup sliced strawberries
- 1 cup raspberries
- 1 cup blueberries
- 1/2 cup sugar
- 1/2 cup fresh orange juice
- 2 cups heavy whipping cream

Directions:

1. Mix sugar, orange juice, and rind (if using) in a small pan.
2. Bring to a boil, stirring to dissolve the sugar.
3. Simmer for approximately 10 minutes without stirring.
4. Cool Syrup.
5. Whip cream into medium peaks.
6. Fold orange syrup into the whipped cream.
7. Serve with berries.
8. For ordinary cream, add 1 tsp vanilla and 2-3 Tbsp powdered sugar (adjust to taste) and whisk until soft peaks form.

Pumpkin Spice Smoothie

Prep time: 5 minutes.
Total Time: 5 minutes.
Servings:2

Ingredients:

- 1/2 cup pumpkin puree.
- One frozen ripe banana.
- 1 cup apple pieces (skin on or off) and 1/2 cup plain Greek yogurt.
- 1/3 cup almond milk (or milk of your choice)
- 1 tablespoon maple syrup.
- 1 teaspoon vanilla.
- 1/2 teaspoon pumpkin pie spice.
- 1/4 teaspoon cinnamon.
- 1/2 cup of ice.

Directions:

1. Place all ingredients in a blender and pulse until smooth and creamy. If the smoothie is too thick, add more milk or water until you reach the desired consistency. Enjoy!

Carrot Apple Delight

Prep time: 8 minutes.
Cook time: 0 minutes.
Total time: 8 minutes.
Servings:2

Ingredients:

- 1 apple, peeled, cored and diced
- Two carrots, peeled and sliced
- One ripe banana.
- 1 cup of unsweetened almond milk.
- 1 teaspoon cinnamon.
- $\frac{1}{2}$ teaspoon lemon juice
- 1/2 cup ice cubes.

Directions:

2. Put the apple, carrots, and banana in a high-speed blender and blend until smooth.
3. Add the remaining ingredients and continue to combine.
4. If necessary, add more almond milk to achieve the desired consistency.
5. Pour into two glasses and serve immediately.

Creamy Chicken Soup

Prep time: 20 minutes.
Cook Time: 25 minutes.
Serves: 6

Ingredients:

- 2 tablespoons olive oil.
- 1 small yellow onion, chopped, approximately 1 cup.
- 1 medium carrot, chopped; 3/4 cup
- 2 diced celery ribs ($\frac{3}{4}$ cup).
- 3 garlic cloves, minced
- 1/4 cup unsalted butter, 4 tablespoons.
- 1/4 cup all-purpose flour.
- 4 cups chicken stock or broth
- 1 cup milk (ideally whole milk).
- 1/2 tsp sea salt, and more to taste
- 1/4 teaspoon of freshly cracked black pepper.
- 1 tablespoon minced fresh dill
- 3 cups shredded cooked chicken from a rotisserie or two large chicken breasts poached in water.
- 1/3 cup grated fresh Parmesan cheese.
- 4 green onions, chopped for garnish.

Directions:

1. Heat olive oil in a large stockpot on medium heat. Once the oil is gleaming, add the onions, carrots, and celery and simmer for 8-10 minutes, or until the carrots and celery begin to soften. Cook until the garlic is aromatic, about 1 minute longer.

2. Add butter to the pan. Once the butter is sizzling, add the flour and whisk until a thick paste forms, about 1 minute. Slowly add the chicken stock while stirring, and bring to a boil over high heat. Once the soup is boiling, reduce the heat and simmer for about 5 minutes, or until the carrots and celery are soft and the soup has thickened.

3. Combine milk, salt, pepper, dill, chicken, and Parmesan cheese. Stir thoroughly. Allow to boil for a few minutes longer, until the chicken is cooked through and the parmesan is fully absorbed.

4. Garnish the soup with green onions and additional Parmesan if preferred.

Tomato Bisque

Prep:5minutes
Cook:15minutes
Total:20minutes
Servings:4

Ingredients:

- 2 tablespoons minced garlic
- 2 tablespoons butter.
- 2 tablespoons all-purpose flour.
- 4 cups chicken broth.
- 14 ounces mashed tomatoes
- 1/4 teaspoon paprika.
- 2 teaspoons garlic salt (with parsley flakes)
- 1 teaspoon basil.

- 1 cup of half & half.

Directions:

1. In a medium saucepan, cook garlic in butter for 1 minute. Then, whisk in the flour until well combined.
2. Pour in the chicken broth gradually. Stir in the tomatoes, paprika, garlic salt, and basil until thoroughly combined.
3. Bring the pot to a boil, then cook for about 2 minutes, or until thickened.
4. Puree the soup in a blender until you get the desired consistency. You will have to perform this in batches.
5. Pour the pureed soup into a serving bowl and mix in the heavy cream. Season with salt and pepper. Garnish with cream and fresh basil.

Fruit & Yogurt Parfait

Prep time: 5 minutes.
Total time: 5 minutes.
Servings:2

Ingredients:

- 1 cup yogurt Natural or Greek yogurt, or a vegan substitute like coconut yogurt, soy yogurt, or almond yogurt
- 1/2 cup granola - nut-free, gluten-free, low-sugar, high-fiber, or high-protein - your choice!
- 1/2 cup strawberries or any fruit of your choice. Peach, nectarine, plum, various berries, pomegranate, and banana
- 1/4 cup blueberries.

* 1 kiwi
* 1/4 cup strawberry sauce or syrup, jams and jellies, etc.

Directions:

1. If you intend to use any homemade ingredients (such as yogurt, granola, or sauce), prepare them first.
2. To make the parfaits, alternating layers of granola, yogurt, sauce, and fruit (1-2 tbsp each) until the glasses/jars are filled. Then, enjoy!

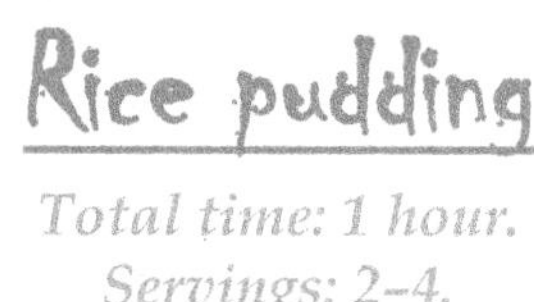

Rice pudding

Total time: 1 hour.
Servings: 2-4.

Ingredients:

* 3/4 cup medium-grained rice or 3/4 cup long-grained rice.
* 1 1/2 cups water.
* 1/4 teaspoon salt (heaping)
* 4 cups of full milk (I used 2%).
* 1/2 cup sugar.
* 1/2 teaspoon vanilla cinnamon.

Directions:

1. Bring rice, water, and salt to boil over medium-high heat.
2. Cover and simmer until water is absorbed, about 15 minutes.
3. Stir in milk and sugar and cook for 30-40 minutes over medium heat, stirring regularly, especially near the end.

4. The pudding is ready when the rice and milk combine into a thick, porridge-like consistency.
5. Avoid overcooking to ensure the pudding remains creamy after cooling.
6. Remove from heat and add vanilla.
7. Transfer into a basin or cups.
8. Optional: Sprinkle cinnamon on top.
9. If you do not want skin, cover the surface directly with plastic wrap.
10.   COOL. And enjoy

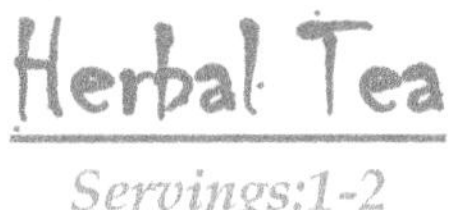

Herbal Tea

Servings:1-2

Ingredients:

- 1 ounce of Chamomile flowers
- 1 ounce of peppermint leaves.
- 1/4-ounce dried ginger root.
- 1/4 ounce of fennel seeds.
- 1/4-ounce dried orange peel

Directions:

1. In a glass jar, combine chamomile flowers, peppermint leaves, dried ginger root, fennel seeds, and dried orange peel. Make sure they're well blended.
2. To prepare a cup of tea, steep 2 to 3 tablespoons in boiling water for 10 minutes, as instructed above.
3. Drink this tummy tea to relieve an upset stomach.

Consume olive oil, avocado, nuts, and seeds. These fats reduce inflammation and promote overall digestive health.

Lunch Recipes

Chicken with Carrot Purée

Ingredients:

- 6 boneless, skin-on chicken breasts pounded to $\frac{3}{4}$" thickness.
- 16 tablespoons (1 cup) olive oil.
- salt to taste
- freshly ground black pepper to taste.
- 4 cups chicken broth.
- Cut 2 pounds of carrots into 1/4" rounds.
- One big white onion, minced
- 1 $\frac{1}{2}$ cup fresh orange juice.
- 4 tablespoons unsalted butter.
- 2 peeled and segmented oranges
- $\frac{3}{4}$ cup plus 2 teaspoons.
- 2 teaspoons sherry vinegar.
- 3 ounces of dandelion greens (may substitute arugula, watercress, or baby spinach leaves).
- $\frac{3}{4}$ cup pitted oil-cured black olives, roughly diced.
- 2 finely sliced shallots

Directions:

1. Place the chicken in a dish and sprinkle with three tablespoons of olive oil. Season with salt and pepper. Set aside. In a 6-quart pan, bring the broth to a boil over medium-high heat. Cook carrots until soft, about 15-20 minutes. Drain. In a 4-quart pot, heat 8 tablespoons (1/2 cup) of olive oil over high heat. Cook until the onions are tender, about 4 to 5 minutes.

Add the carrots and simmer for 6 to 8 minutes. Puree in a food processor with 2 tablespoons oil. Season with salt and pepper, and keep heated.

2. In a 2-quart pan, bring the orange juice to a boil over medium-high heat. Simmer for 12 to 15 minutes, or until reduced by half. Add the butter, whisk, and season with the salt and pepper. Add the orange segments and put aside the sauce.

3. Preheat oven to 400 °F. Preheat a grill pan to medium-high heat. Working in batches, fry the chicken until crisp, 8 to 10 minutes. Place chicken, skin side up, on a baking sheet. Brush with 3/4 cup harissa. Bake for approximately 8 minutes.

4. In a bowl, combine the remaining oil, harissa, and sherry vinegar. Add the greens, olives, and shallots, and toss. Divide the carrot purée across six plates, then top with salad and a chicken breast. Spoon the sauce over each.

Lentil Soup

Prep time: 10 minutes.
Cook Time: 45 minutes.
Total time: 55 minutes.
Servings: 4

Ingredients:

- 1/4 cup extra virgin olive oil.
- 1 medium yellow or white onion, diced.
- Peel and cut 2 carrots. Press or mince 4 garlic cloves.
- 2 tablespoons ground cumin
- 1 teaspoon of curry powder.

- $\frac{1}{2}$ teaspoon dried thyme.
- 1 large can (28 oz.) Diced tomatoes, lightly drained
- 1 cup brown or green lentils, cleaned and rinsed
- Combine 4 cups veggie broth and 2 cups water.
- 1 teaspoon salt, add more to taste.
- A pinch of red pepper flakes.
- freshly ground black pepper to taste.
- 1 cup chopped fresh collard greens or kale with tough ribs removed.
- 1 to 2 tablespoons lemon juice ($\frac{1}{2}$ to 1 full lemon) to taste.

Directions:

1. Heat olive oil in a large Dutch oven or saucepan over medium heat. One-fourth cup of olive oil may seem excessive, but it gives a delightful richness and heartiness to this healthful soup.
2. Cook the chopped onion and carrot in the oil until softened and translucent, about 5 minutes. Stir frequently.
3. Combine garlic, cumin, curry powder, and thyme. Cook for about 30 seconds or until aromatic, stirring regularly. Pour in the drained diced tomatoes and simmer for a few more minutes, stirring frequently, to intensify the taste.
4. Pour in lentils, broth, and water. Combine 1 teaspoon salt and a pinch of red pepper flakes. Season generously with fresh ground black pepper. Bring the mixture to a boil, then partially cover and decrease heat to a slow simmer. Cook for 25–30

minutes, or until the lentils are cooked but still maintain their shape.

5. Add 2 cups of soup to a blender. Secure the lid, cover it with a tea towel to protect your hand from steam, and purée the soup until smooth. Pour the pureed soup back into the pot. (Alternatively, use an immersion blender to mix a part of the soup.

6. Cook for 5 minutes more, or until greens are softened to your preference. Take the pot off of the burner and squeeze in one tablespoon of lemon juice. Taste and season with extra salt, pepper, and/or lemon juice until the flavors are bursting. For a hotter soup, add an extra pinch or two of red pepper flakes.

7. Serve hot. Leftovers can be stored in the refrigerator for up to four days or frozen for several months.

Creamy Spinach Soup

Prep Time:10 mins
Cook Time: 35 minutes.
Total Time: 45 minutes.
Servings:5

Ingredients:

- 1-pound frozen chopped spinach, thawed.
- 2 glasses of water.
- 4 teaspoons chicken bouillon granules.
- $\frac{1}{2}$ cup chopped onion, $\frac{1}{4}$ teaspoon garlic powder.
- $\frac{1}{4}$ cup butter
- 1/4 cup all-purpose flour

- Combine 3 cups of half-and-half
- salt and pepper to taste.

Directions:

1. Combine spinach, water, bouillon, onion, and garlic powder in a large pot over medium-high heat. Bring to a boil, then reduce to medium-low and cook until the onion is soft.
2. In a small saucepan, melt the butter and mix in the flour until smooth. Cook for two minutes. Slowly stir in the half-and-half, mixing until smooth. Pour the cream mixture into the spinach soup and simmer for 10 minutes, or until thickened. Season to taste with salt and pepper.

Turkey and rice porridge

Preparation time: 20 minutes
Cook time: 45 minutes.
Total time: 1 hour, 5 minutes.
Servings:8

Ingredients:

- 12 cups turkey stock, plus a little extra to dilute (2.8 liters).
- 2 cups of rinsed and drained rice (400g)
- 2-inch ginger, peeled and crushed
- 12 red dates (rinsed, soaking for 20 minutes, and drained)
- 3 cups (450 grams) Turkey meat
- Salt to taste.
- Grind pepper to taste.

- $\frac{1}{4}$ cup goji berries, rinsed and steeped for 10 minutes before draining. (30g)

For Garnish:

- Thinly sliced green onion
- Season with pepper and sesame oil.
- Soy sauce

Directions:

1. Add turkey stock to a big pot. Combine rice, ginger, and red dates. Turn on the stove and bring to a boil. When the stock comes to a boil, remove the lid and add the turkey, salt, and pepper. Reduce the heat and let it simmer for about 30 minutes.
2. Add goji berries and simmer for another 15 minutes. If the porridge becomes too thick, add $\frac{1}{2}$ cup water to adjust the consistency.
3. Serve immediately in individual bowls after removing from heat. Sprinkle with green onions and pepper, then drizzle with a few drops of sesame oil and soy sauce.

Quinoa Vegetable Soup

Prep time: 30 minutes.
Cook Time: 45 minutes.
Total time: 1 hour 15 minutes.
Servings:6

Ingredients:

- 2 tablespoons olive oil.
- 2 tablespoons butter
- 1 chopped onion and $\frac{1}{2}$ cup diced carrot.
- 1/2 cup chopped celery.
- 1 clove garlic, minced
- 2 (32-ounce) cartons of Chicken broth
- 1 (28-ounce) can crushed tomatoes
- 2 teaspoons of dried parsley.
- 1 teaspoon dried basil.
- 1 bay leaf and 1 pinch dried thyme.
- 2 cups shredded cabbage.
- 1 (15-ounce) can of light red kidney beans, drained.
- $\frac{1}{2}$ cup quinoa
- 1/2 cup grated Parmesan cheese (optional)

Directions:

1. Heat olive oil and butter in a big saucepan or Dutch oven on medium heat. Cook and stir in the onion, carrot, celery, and garlic until they are cooked, about 3 to 5 minutes. Bring to a boil and stir in the chicken broth, tomatoes, parsley, basil, bay leaf, and thyme. Reduce the heat to a simmer for about 5 minutes, or until well heated.

2. Add cabbage, kidney beans, and quinoa to the soup. Cover and cook until the quinoa is cooked, about 30 minutes. Garnish each serving with parmesan cheese.

Creamy salmon bisque

Prep time: 15 minutes.
Cook time: 20 minutes.
Total: 35 minutes.
4 servings.

Ingredients:

- 6 tablespoons (3 ounces) of unsalted butter.
- 1 tablespoon grated onion, 5 tablespoons all-purpose flour.
- Use 1 medium bay leaf and 3/4 cup low-sodium or unsalted chicken broth or stock.
- 1/2 cup of dry white wine.
- 1 tablespoon of tomato paste.
- 1 (7.5-ounce) can of salmon with juices
- 1 cup half-and-half or whole milk.
- Kosher salt (to taste)
- freshly ground black pepper to taste.
- For optional garnish, add roasted red pepper strips, sour cream, olive oil, croutons, and chopped fresh parsley

Directions:

1. Gather all ingredients.
2. Melt butter in a medium skillet. Add shredded onion and sauté for 4 to 5 minutes until tender.

3. Add flour to the butter and onion mixture. Cook, stirring regularly, for 2 minutes. Add the bay leaf and gradually incorporate the broth. Cook, stirring, until thick and smooth.
4. Add wine and simmer on low heat for 10 minutes. Discard the bay leaf.
5. Stir in tomato paste, fish, and liquids. Blend in batches until smooth, then return to saucepan. Alternatively, use a hand blender to purée the bisque right in the pot.
6. Add half-and-half and season with salt and pepper to taste.
7. Optional garnishes include roasted red pepper slices, croutons, sour cream, or fresh parsley.
8. Enjoy.

Sweet Potato Puree

Prep Time:15 mins
Cook Time: 45 minutes.
Total time: 1 hour,
Servings: 8

Ingredients:

- pierce 3 pounds of whole sweet potatoes with a fork and season with salt and ground black pepper to taste.
- $\frac{1}{2}$ cup buttermilk
- 1/2 cup whole milk.
- 6 tablespoons butter, softened

Directions:

1. Turn the oven's temperature up to 425 degrees Fahrenheit (220°C). Arrange a rack in the upper center position of the oven. Line a baking tray with aluminum foil.

2. Bake potatoes on a prepared pan in a preheated oven for 45-60 minutes. Peel once cold enough to handle.

3. Puree peeled potatoes in a food processor until smooth. Season with salt and pepper. With the engine running, gradually add buttermilk and milk through the feeder tube, followed by butter. Continue processing until silky smooth.

Tomato Basil Soup

Prep Time: 15minutes mins
Cook Time: 1 hour, 30 minutes.
Servings: 6 to 8.

Ingredients:

- To prepare, halve $2\frac{1}{2}$ pounds of Roma tomatoes and divide $\frac{1}{4}$ cup of extra-virgin olive oil evenly.
- Chop one medium yellow onion and $\frac{1}{3}$ cup carrots.
- Combine 4 chopped garlic cloves with 3 cups of vegetable broth.
- 1 tablespoon of balsamic vinegar.
- 1 teaspoon of thyme leaves.
- 1 loose-packed cup of basil leaves, extra for garnish.
- Sea salt, freshly ground black pepper.

Directions:

1. Preheat oven to 350°F and prepare a large baking sheet with parchment paper. Place the tomatoes cut-side up on the baking pan, drizzle with 2 tablespoons olive oil, and season

with salt and pepper. Roast for an hour, or until the edges begin to shrivel but the insides remain moist.

2. Heat the remaining 2 tablespoons of olive oil in a large pot over medium heat. Cook the onions, carrots, garlic, and $\frac{1}{2}$ teaspoon salt until tender, about 8 minutes. Stir in the tomatoes, vegetable broth, vinegar, and thyme leaves, then cook for 20 minutes.
3. Once cooled, transfer the soup to a blender, working in batches as needed. Blend until smooth. Add the basil and pulse to mix.
4. Top the soup with basil leaves and serve with crusty bread.

Zucchini Potato Soup

Prep Time: 25 minutes.
Cook Time: 35 minutes.
Total Time: 1 hour.
Servings:8

Ingredients:

- 2 tablespoons butter
- 2 onions, chopped.
- Two potatoes, peeled and diced
- 8 sliced zucchini, $\frac{1}{2}$ teaspoon dried basil, $\frac{1}{4}$ teaspoon dry thyme, and $\frac{1}{4}$ teaspoon dried rosemary
- $\frac{1}{4}$ teaspoon ground white pepper.
- 4 cups chicken broth.
- 1 cup whole milk.
- $\frac{1}{4}$ cup dry potato flakes (optional).

- 1 tablespoon of soy sauce.
- 4 teaspoons of chopped fresh dill weed.

Directions:

1. In a large skillet, melt butter over medium heat and toss in onion. Cook and stir for 5 minutes, or until the onion softens and becomes translucent. Cook and mix in the diced potato, zucchini, basil, thyme, rosemary, and white pepper until the zucchini softens, about 5 minutes.
2. Bring broth to a simmer and cook until potatoes are tender approximately 15 minutes.
3. Puree soup with an immersion blender until it's smooth. Stir in milk and heat through without boiling. To thin out the soup, stir in some potato flakes. Season to taste with soy sauce and serve with dill weed.

Cauliflower Cheese Soup

Preparation: 10 minutes.
Servings: 6-8.

Ingredients:

- A chunk of butter.
- One big onion, coarsely sliced
- 1 large cauliflower (approximately 900g/2lb), trimmed leaves and sliced into florets.
- 1 peeled potato, cut into bits
- 700ml vegetable stock (using a cube is fine)

- 400 ml milk
- 100g mature cheddar, diced

Directions:

1. In a large pot, melt the butter. Add the onion and simmer for about 5 minutes, stirring frequently. Combine the cauliflower, potato, stock, milk, and seasonings. Bring to a boil, then reduce heat and simmer for 30 minutes, or until the cauliflower is soft and the potato is almost collapsed.
2. Use a food processor or a potato masher to create a creamy, thick soup. If serving in mugs, add extra milk to thin it out slightly. You can prepare up to two days ahead of time, chill, cover, and store in the refrigerator until needed, or freeze for up to a month. When ready to serve, heat through, spoon into cups or bowls, top with cheese slices, and swirl before eating.

Dinner Recipes

Vegetable and Tofu Soup

Prep Time:35 mins
Additional Time: 2 hours.
Total time: 2 hours, 35 minutes.
Servings:4

Ingredients:

- 1 (12-ounce) box of extra-firm tub-style tofu (fresh bean curd), drained and cut into 3/4-inch cubes.
- 2 tablespoons olive oil.
- 1 teaspoon dry Italian seasoning, crushed
- nonstick cooking spray
- 2 cups of reduced-sodium chicken broth
- One (14.5 ounces) can of no-undrained diced tomatoes with basil, garlic, and oregano, seasoned with salt
- 3 cups of sliced fresh button mushrooms (8 ounces).
- ½ cup fresh or frozen peas, thawed. 1-inch slices of asparagus
- 1/2 cup chopped roasted red sweet pepper.
- ⅓ cup oil-packed dried tomatoes, finely chopped, and ¼ cup sliced green olives.
- One pinch of shredded parmesan cheese

Directions:

1. Set tofu in a resealable plastic bag on a shallow dish. Combine oil and Italian seasoning. Seal the bag and turn to coat the tofu. Marinate in the refrigerator for 2-4 hours.
2. Coat a 5- to 6-quart Dutch oven in cooking spray and heat on medium-high. Add the undrained tofu and heat for 5 to 8 minutes, stirring once, until browned.

3. Combine the broth and canned tomatoes. Bring to a boil. Add the mushrooms, peas, and asparagus; decrease the heat. Simmer for 5–7 minutes, or until the vegetables are soft. Add the sweet pepper, dried tomatoes, and olives; heat through. If preferred, top each serving with cheese.

Mashed Potato and Turkey Soup

Preparation: 30 minutes.
Total: 2 hours and 30 minutes.
Servings: 6 - 8.

Ingredients:

- 8 cups chicken broth.
- 1 turkey carcass with all meat removed.
- 1 carrot, halved lengthwise, and 1 carrot, minced
- 1 full stalk celery, 1 chopped stalk, and 1 halved onion.
- Two bay leaves.
- 3 cups of dark turkey flesh.
- 2 garlic cloves, crushed
- 2 tablespoons olive oil.
- 3 cups leftover cooked Thanksgiving side veggies (Brussels sprouts, sweet potatoes, and green beans)
- 1 tablespoon of chopped fresh sage.
- Mashed Potato Polpetti (Patties), for serving, recipe below.
- Mashed potato polpetti (patties):
- 3 cups mashed potatoes.
- Grey salt, freshly ground black pepper.
- 1/2 cup grated Parmesan.

- All-purpose flour for dredging.
- 1/4 cup extra virgin olive oil.
- Leftover gravy for serving.

Directions:

1. Combine chicken broth, turkey, carrots, celery stalk, onion halves, and 1 bay leaf in a large stockpot. Bring to a boil, then reduce to a simmer for approximately 1 1/2 hours.
2. Dice turkey meat. Make sure the meat pieces are no bigger than a soupspoon. (If making the soup the next day, make sure to keep any leftover turkey meat in an airtight container before refrigerating. Top with 1 or 2 ladles of broth to keep the meat juicy.
3. Before filtering the soup, use tongs to remove the major bones and carcasses. Strain the broth through a strainer lined with damp cheesecloth. Discard the solids. Transfer the soup to a bowl immersed in ice water, which will cool it rapidly and keep it fresher for longer. This can be done the night before and kept in the fridge until the following day.
4. In a large soup pot, cook garlic in olive oil over medium heat. Allow to brown slightly, approximately 3 minutes. Combine the minced carrots, celery, and onions. Sweat over medium-low heat for 7 or 8 minutes, until softened.
5. Dice leftover Thanksgiving vegetables. Add the sage to the soup pot, along with the turkey broth and the last bay leaf. Bring to a simmer. When the soup has reached a simmer, add the Brussels sprouts, green beans, and cubed turkey meat.

Bring it back to a simmer. Finally, place the sweet potatoes in the center and gently push them down. Turn off the heat and cover. Allow to sit and steam for 5–7 minutes. Simmer for 5 minutes more, then serve with the Mashed Potato Polpetti.

6. Reseason potatoes with salt and pepper. Stir in the cheese. To create a mold, line a mayonnaise or peanut butter lid with plastic wrap. Pack the potato mixture into the lid, then unwrap and place the patty on a baking pan. You can refrigerate them covered in plastic wrap until the next day, or cook them right away.

7. To cook, coat the patties in flour. Heat the oil in a nonstick skillet over medium-high heat. Dredge the patties in flour once more just before frying them.

8. Cook the patties in batches to avoid crowding the oil. Cook for approximately 5 minutes or until the underside is golden brown. Flip and brown the opposite side. Remove from the skillet and let drain on paper towels. Serve hot with any leftover gravy. Makes six servings.

9. This recipe from Food Network Kitchens has been modified for optimal results following additional testing.

Creamy Asparagus Soup

Prep Time: 20 minutes
Cook Time: 25 minutes.
Total time 45 minutes.
Servings:4

Ingredients:

- 1 ½ pounds asparagus, trimmed and rinsed.
- 1 tablespoon butter, 1 tiny diced onion.
- 1 clove garlic, minced
- 2 ¼ cups chicken broth, not low sodium.
- Salt and black pepper to taste.
- 1/2 cup heavy cream or to taste.
- ½ teaspoon lemon juice. Optional: Serve with fresh parmesan cheese.

Directions:

1. Cut asparagus into ½ inch pieces.
2. Cook onion and garlic in butter on medium heat until soft. Cook for a further 5 minutes after adding the asparagus.
3. Stir in broth, salt, and pepper. Cover and boil for 10-15 minutes, or until the asparagus softens.
4. Using a hand blender, mix the soup until smooth. Stir in the cream and lemon juice.
5. Adjust seasoning with salt and pepper as needed.

<h1 style="text-align:center">Beet and Carrot Puree</h1>

Ingredients:

- 1 medium carrot
- 1/2 medium-sized beetroot

Directions:

1. Wash carrots and beetroot. Peel and cut equally.
2. Steam or pressure cook carrot and beetroot chunks until soft.
3. Use a spoon or fork to check if the pieces are cooked through. You should be able to cut the pieces easily.
4. Let the cooked vegetables cool down. Now, transfer them to a grinder jar or food processor and pulse until smooth. To thin out the puree, use any remaining cooking liquid or hot water.
5. Warm the purée and serve immediately.

<h1 style="text-align:center">Egg Drop Soup</h1>

Prep Time:5 mins
Cook time: 10 minutes.
Total Time: 15 minutes.
Servings:1

Ingredients:

- 1 cup chicken broth, $\frac{1}{4}$ teaspoon soy sauce.
- $\frac{1}{4}$ teaspoon sesame oil
- Two teaspoons of water (optional)
- 1 teaspoon of cornstarch (optional)
- Beat 1 large egg and add 1 drop of yellow food coloring (optional).

- $\frac{1}{2}$ teaspoon of ground white pepper (optional)
- 1/8 teaspoon salt (optional)
- 1 teaspoon of chopped fresh chives.

Directions:

1. Gather all the ingredients.
2. In a small saucepan over medium heat, combine the chicken broth, soy sauce, and sesame oil. Bring to a boil.
3. In a separate bowl, combine water and cornstarch; stir until dissolved; pour into boiling broth. Stir in the food coloring.
4. Slowly pour in the beaten egg while stirring frequently; season with white pepper and salt.
5. Serve hot and garnished with fresh chives. Enjoy!

Cucumber Avocado Gazpacho

Preparation time: 10 minutes.
Total time is 10 minutes.
Serves: 4 cups

Ingredients:

- 2 cucumbers (a large green type of preference).
- 1 avocado, medium-sized
- $\frac{1}{2}$ cup cilantro or fresh basil.
- 1/2 cup parsley, curly or flat leaf.
- 1/2 cup sour cream, yogurt, or coconut cream.
- 2 tablespoons lime juice (about the juice of one lime)

- ¼ red onion (or 3 green onions, green half alone for low FODMAP)
- 1 clove garlic (omit for low FODMAP)
- 1/2 cup olive oil (or garlic-infused olive oil for low FODMAP)
- 1 tablespoon sherry vinegar (you can also use white wine, champagne, or apple cider vinegar).
- 1 teaspoon sea salt (to taste)
- Add ¼ teaspoon pepper (or to taste).
- ¼ teaspoon cumin (optional).

Directions:

1. Peel and remove seeds from cucumber. This removes any bitterness that they may have added to the soup.
2. Remove large stems from parsley and cilantro and wash thoroughly to remove contaminants. I prefer to use a little salad spinner for this.
3. Combine all ingredients in a blender and process until smooth.
4. Taste and adjust seasonings as necessary.
5. Refrigerate until ready to serve.

Broccoli Potato Mash

Preparation Time: 10 minutes
Cook time: 10 minutes.
Total time: 20 minutes
Servings:4-6

Ingredients:

- 1 pound Yukon Gold potatoes, diced (peeled if desired).
- 2 cups broccoli florets, roughly chopped.

- 1 tablespoon of unsalted butter (or olive oil).
- 2 tablespoons sour cream.
- 1/4 to 1/2 teaspoon salt.

Directions:

1. Place potatoes in a medium-large saucepan and cover with 2 inches of cold water. Bring to a boil, then reduce heat and simmer for approximately 6 minutes, or until almost soft.
2. Simmer until broccoli and potatoes are tender but not mushy, approximately 4 minutes.
3. Drain through a colander.
4. Combine butter, sour cream, and salt. Mash with a potato masher until the mixture is as lumpy or smooth as you prefer.

Part II: Low Fiber Diet

In this section, a low-fiber or low-residue diet is recommended during Diverticulitis recovery.

These are foods with a low fiber and residue content. This temporary healing diet, sometimes called a soft diet, includes the following foods:

Starchy foods: Potatoes (no skin), white rice, White bread

a) **Dairy:** milk and cottage cheese.
b) **Protein:** Eggs, fish, lean poultry, yogurt, gelatin
c) **Fruit:** applesauce, canned or cooked fruit, fruit juice (without pulp)
d) **Vegetables:** well-cooked.
e) **Liquids:** broth, ice pops.

Staying hydrated is essential for proper bowel movement. Drink plenty of water throughout the day to help prevent constipation and maintain regularity.

Breakfast Recipes

Creamy scrambled eggs

Ingredients:

- 1/2 tbsp butter.
- Four big eggs.
- 1/8 teaspoon kosher salt (or more to taste)

Directions:

1. Melt the butter in a medium nonstick pan over medium-low heat.
2. Crack the eggs into a bowl, add a touch of salt, and whisk until thoroughly combined.
3. When the butter begins to boil, throw in the eggs and immediately swirl in small circles around the pan with a silicone spatula, without stopping, until the eggs appear slightly thicker and very small curds develop, which should take around 30 seconds.
4. Change from forming circles to long strokes across the pan until you see larger, creamy curds (approximately 20 seconds).
5. When the eggs are softly set and somewhat runny in places, turn off the heat and let them cook for a few seconds. Give it a final swirl and serve immediately. Serve with an extra sprinkling of salt, a grind of black pepper, and a few fresh chopped herbs (optional).

Fruit and yogurt parfait

Prepare for 5 minutes.
Total time: 5 minutes.
Serves: 3

Ingredients:

- 1 32-ounce carton of whole milk vanilla yogurt.
- 1-pound fresh berries of choice, chopped
- 1 ½ - 2 cups vanilla granola (or your preferred flavor)
- 3 Tablespoons Honey

Directions:

1. Scoop ⅓ cup of yogurt into three glass jars or containers.
2. 1 32-ounce carton of whole milk vanilla yogurt.
3. Sprinkle the berries on top.
4. 1-pound fresh berries of your choice
5. Add the granola, setting aside at least 3 tablespoons.
6. 1 ½ - 2 cups vanilla granola (or your preferred flavor)
7. Divide the remaining yogurt among the parfaits, dolloping some on each.
8. Top each jar with the remaining granola and drizzle with a spoonful of honey.
9. 3 Tablespoons Honey
10. Enjoy immediately, or keep in the fridge for up to 2-3 days.

Oatmeal with Nut Butter

Prep/Total Time: 15 min.
Servings:2

Ingredients:

- 1 3/4 cups of water
- 1/8 teaspoon of salt.
- 1 cup old-fashioned oatmeal
- 2 tablespoons of creamy peanut butter.
- 2 tablespoons honey.
- 2 teaspoons of ground flaxseed.
- 1/2 to 1 teaspoon of ground cinnamon.
- Chopped apple is optional.

Directions:

1. In a small saucepan, heat water and salt till boiling.
2. Stir in the oats and simmer for 5 minutes over medium heat, stirring periodically.
3. Transfer the oats to two bowls. In each bowl, combine half of the peanut butter, honey, flaxseed, cinnamon, and, if preferred, apple.
4. Serve immediately.

Rice Pudding Prep

Time: 5 minutes
Cook: 2 hours.
Serves: 4

Ingredients:

- 100g pudding rice
- Butter,
- 50g sugar.
- 700ml semi-skimmed milk
- a teaspoon of grated nutmeg
- lemon zest (strips).
- 1 bay leaf or strip of lemon zest

Directions:

1. Preheat the oven to 150C/130C fan/gas
2. Wash and drain the rice. Butter an 850ml baking dish, then add the rice and sugar.
3. Stir in the milk. Add the nutmeg and top with the bay leaf or lemon zest.
4. Cook for two hours, or until the pudding wobbles slightly when shaken.

Poached Eggs on Toast

Preparation time: 5 minutes
Cook time: 4 minutes.
Total Time: 9 minutes.

Ingredients:

- Water in a small pot. 1 1/2 inch deep.
- 1 teaspoon white vinegar.
- 1 egg
- Add sea salt
- and freshly cracked pepper to taste.
- One slice of buttered bread.

Directions:

1. In a small saucepan, heat 1 1/2 inches of water and vinegar until simmering.
2. Crack one egg into a small bowl. When the water has reached a simmer, stir it with the bottom of a slotted spoon clockwise to create a swirling motion. Quickly and carefully lower the egg into the water.
3. Cover and switch off the stove. Poach for 3 minutes and 45 seconds, or until the whites are firm but the yolks remain runny. Using a slotted spoon, remove the egg and let it drain slightly over the pan.
4. Place on buttered toast and season with sea salt and cracked pepper to taste. Serve immediately. Enjoy!

Baked apples with cinnamon

Prep time: 10 minutes.
Cook time: 1 hour.
Total time: 1 hour, 10 minutes.
Servings:6

Ingredients:

Apples:

- 6-7 medium to large apples (2 tart-like granny smith
- 4 sweet like Honeycrisp
- 2 tablespoons lemon juice.
- 1 tablespoon coconut oil (optional).
- 2/3 cup coconut sugar (or organic cane sugar // substitute up to half with stevia to taste*)
- 1 ½ teaspoon ground cinnamon
- 3/4 teaspoon freshly grated ginger*
- 1 sprinkle of nutmeg.
- 3 tablespoons cornstarch or arrowroot starch (to thicken the sauce).
- 3 tablespoons fresh apple juice or water.
- 1 pinch of sea salt.

For Serving (Optional):

- Coconut Whipped Cream
- Vanilla Bean Coconut Ice Cream*.

Directions:

1. Preheat oven to 350 degrees F (176 C) and prepare a 9×13-inch (or comparable size) baking dish.

2. Peel and core apples, then quarter and thinly slice lengthwise with a paring knife (see photo). The thinner, the better. Simply try to be consistent so that they cook evenly.

3. Pour into baking dish and sprinkle with lemon juice, coconut oil (optional), coconut sugar, cinnamon, ginger, nutmeg, cornstarch (or arrowroot), apple juice (or water), and salt. Toss to blend. Then, loosely wrap with foil.

4. Bake for 45 minutes, covered. Then, carefully remove the cover and bake for another 10-15 minutes, or until the apples are fork-soft (particularly in the center of the dish) and slightly caramelized (see photo).

5. Serve with coconut whipped cream or vanilla bean coconut ice cream. Best when fresh, but leftovers can be kept covered in the refrigerator for 3-4 days or frozen for up to 1 month. Reheat in the microwave or a 350-degree F (176-degree C) oven (covered) until heated through. If the "caramel" sauce is excessively thick, thin it out with some water.

<u>Scrambled tofu with vegetables</u>

Prep time: 5 minutes.
Cook Time: 5 minutes.
Total Time: 10 minutes.
Servings: 1

Ingredients:

- 4 ounces extra-firm tofu, leafy greens (spinach, kale, mixed greens, or arugula).
- Chop 1/4 cup red or yellow pepper, dice 1/4 avocado, and season with salt and pepper.

Spice Sauce Ingredients:

- Add 1 tsp turmeric, and a dash of cumin, and season with salt and pepper to taste.
- 2 tablespoons water

Directions:

1. Preheat a nonstick pan over medium heat.
2. In a small bowl, combine spices and water to prepare spice sauce while the pan heats up.

3.	Squeeze the water out of the tofu with your hands over the sink. Try to remove as much water as possible.

4.	Using your hands or a fork, crumble the tofu into the pan. Pour the spice sauce over it and mix.

5.	Cook for 2-3 minutes. Transfer to a dish and put aside.

6.	Cook red peppers with oil, salt, and pepper in the same pan for 5 minutes.

7.	Combine cooked red peppers with remaining vegetables in a tofu scramble and enjoy!

Lunch Recipes

Tuna Salad Sandwich

Preparation: 15 minutes.
Total: 15 minutes.
Servings:4

Ingredients:

- 2 cans (6 oz each) of tuna in water, drained
- 1/2 cup chopped celery.
- 1/4 cup chopped onion,
- 1/2 cup mayonnaise or salad dressing.
- 1 teaspoon lemon juice.
- 1/4 teaspoon salt.
- 1/4 teaspoon pepper.
- Eight slices of bread

Directions:

1. In a medium bowl, combine the tuna, celery, onion, mayonnaise, lemon juice, salt, and pepper.
2. Spread the tuna mixture on four slices of bread. Top with the remaining bread slices.

Mac & Cheese

Prep time: 10 minutes.
Cook Time: 15 minutes.
Total Time: 25 minutes.
Servings:4

Ingredients:

- 1 (8-oz) box elbow macaroni
- Add $\frac{1}{4}$ cup butter and $\frac{1}{4}$ cup all-purpose flour.
- $\frac{1}{2}$ teaspoon salt to taste.

- ground black pepper to taste.
- 2 cups milk.
- 2 cups shredded cheddar cheese.

Directions:

1. Heat a big saucepan of lightly salted water to a boil. Cook elbow macaroni in boiling water for 8 minutes, tossing regularly, until it is cooked through yet firm to the biting.
2. At the same time, melt the butter in a saucepan over medium heat.
3. Stir in the flour, salt, and pepper until smooth, about 5 minutes.
4. Pour in the milk gently, stirring continually. Continue to heat and stir until the mixture is smooth and bubbling, about 5 minutes, keeping the milk from burning.
5. Stir in the Cheddar cheese until melted, about 2 to 4 minutes.
6. Drain the macaroni and fold it into the cheese sauce until it is covered.
7. Serve hot, and enjoy!

Egg Drop Soup

Prep time: 5 minutes.
Cook time: 10 minutes.
Total time: 15 minutes.
Serving size: 6 cups of soup

Ingredients:

- 4 cups high-quality chicken or veggie stock.

- 2 tablespoons cornstarch
- 2 teaspoons ground ginger.
- 1 teaspoon of garlic powder.
- 1/8 teaspoon of white pepper.
- Three huge eggs.
- 1 teaspoon toasted sesame oil
- fine sea salt, and cracked black pepper to taste.
- thinly sliced green onions.

Directions:

1. Prepare the broth. In a medium saucepan, combine stock (chilled or room temperature), cornstarch, ginger, garlic powder, and white pepper. Whisk until smooth. Cook over high heat, stirring regularly, until the stock reaches a simmer.
2. Whisk the eggs. Meanwhile, combine the eggs and egg whites in a small measuring cup or basin. (I prefer using a measuring cup for pouring.)
3. Stir in egg ribbons. When the soup reaches a simmer, use a whisk or two chopsticks to swirl it in a circular motion to form a vortex. Then, while continuing to stir, slowly pour the whisked eggs into the soup in a very thin stream, creating egg ribbons.
4. Season. Remove the pan from the heat. Stir in the sesame oil until thoroughly blended. Season to taste with salt and white pepper, and if necessary, add a dash or two more sesame oil. Depending on the brand of chicken stock, this soup may require an additional $\frac{1}{2}$ to 1 teaspoon of fine sea salt.

5. Serve. Serve immediately, topped with plenty of green onions and a twist of black pepper.

Chicken Noodle Soup

Preparation: 5 minutes.
Cook:35mins
Total:40mins

Ingredients:

- Two tablespoons of butter, chicken fat, or olive oil
- One large onion, chopped.
- Two big carrots, chopped.
- 2 celery stalks, diced (optional).
- A heaping tablespoon of minced garlic (4 cloves)
- Two bay leaves.
- 3 sprigs fresh thyme, or use 1/2 teaspoon of dried thyme.
- 1-pound skinless, boneless chicken thighs (four or five)
- 8 cups of low-sodium chicken stock or broth, or homemade stock
- 5 oz egg noodles (or pasta of your choice)
- Add salt and pepper to taste.
- 1/4 cup fresh parsley, finely chopped
- Water or additional stock, as needed.

Directions:

1. In a big pot or Dutch oven over medium heat, melt the butter. Combine the onion, carrots, and celery. Cook, stirring every few minutes, until the veggies soften, about 5 to 6 minutes.

2. Stir in the garlic, bay leaves, and thyme. Cook for approximately 1 minute, moving the garlic around the pan.
3. Add the chicken stock and bring to a moderate simmer. Taste the soup, then season with salt and pepper. Depending on the stock, you may need to add one or more teaspoons of salt.
4. Immerse the chicken thighs in the soup so that the stock covers them. Bring the soup back to a low simmer, then partially cover with a lid and cook, stirring occasionally, until the chicken thighs are cooked through, about 20 minutes.
5. If the broth appears to be running low during this time, add a dash of stock or a little water. Set the heat to medium-low.
6. Move the cooked chicken to a plate. Stir the noodles into the broth and cook for 6 to 10 minutes, depending on the type of noodles.
7. While the noodles cook, cut the chicken into strips or cubes. Return the chicken to the stove and taste the soup again for spice. Adjust with additional salt and pepper as needed. Stir in the parsley and serve.

Hummus & Veggie Wraps

Preparation time: 5 minutes.
Total time: 5 minutes.
Servings: One wrap.

Ingredients:

- One flavored wrap or tortilla (I used spinach)
- ⅓ Cup Hummus
- 2 slices of cucumber, cut lengthwise

- A handful of fresh spinach leaves.
- Sliced tomatoes (depending on their size)
- $\frac{1}{4}$ avocado, sliced
- Fresh alfalfa or broccoli sprouts.
- Fresh microgreens.
- basil leaves if desired.

Directions:

1. Spread the hummus on the bottom ⅓ of the wrap, leaving about $\frac{1}{2}$ inch from the bottom edge and spreading out to the sides.
2. Layer cucumber, spinach, tomato, avocado, sprouts, microgreens, and basil.
3. Fold the wrap tightly like a burrito, tucking in all the veggies with the initial roll and rolling hard till the finish. Cut in half and enjoy.

Eating smaller, more frequent meals throughout the day will assist to avoid overloading your digestive system and reduce diverticulitis symptoms.

Dinner Recipes

Baked salmon with lemon & herbs

Prep time: 5 minutes.
Cook time: 15 minutes.
Total time:20 minutes.
Servings:4

Ingredients:

- 3-4 salmon fillets
- 2 tablespoons melted butter
- Two medium lemons.
- 1/4 cup roughly chopped fresh herbs (thyme, oregano, rosemary, parsley, or basil are all suitable)
- Minced garlic (3 cloves) with kosher salt and black pepper.

Directions:

1. Preheat oven to 425 degrees Fahrenheit. Line a rimmed baking sheet with parchment paper and set the salmon filets on top, skin-side down.
2. Brush the melted butter evenly over the filets.
3. Juice one lemon, then add the chopped herbs and minced garlic. Add a liberal amount of salt and pepper. Spoon the mixture evenly over the salmon filets. Thinly slice the remaining lemon and arrange pieces on top of each filet.
4. Place the fish in the oven and cook for 10-14 minutes. Cooking time will vary depending on the thickness of the fish.. For tender yet safe salmon, use an instant-read thermometer and remove it when the thickest part of the filets reaches 145

degrees Fahrenheit. When the salmon is opaque and readily flaked with a fork, you know it's done.

5. Garnish with more sprigs of fresh herbs and lemon wedges, if preferred. Serve, and enjoy!

Chicken Stir-Fry

Prep time: 20 minutes.
Cook time: 20 minutes.
Total Time: 40 minutes.
Servings:6

Ingredients:

- 4 cups of water.
- 2 cups white rice.
- ⅔ cup soy sauce.
- $\frac{1}{4}$ cup brown sugar
- 1 tablespoon cornstarch and 1 tablespoon minced fresh ginger.
- 1 tablespoon of minced garlic.
- $\frac{1}{4}$ teaspoon red pepper flakes.
- Three skinless, boneless chicken breast halves, thinly sliced
- Two teaspoons of sesame oil, split
- 1 head broccoli, broken into florets.
- 1 onion, chopped into large bits
- 1 cup chopped carrots.
- 1 (8 ounces) can of sliced water chestnuts, drained.
- One green bell pepper, sliced into matchsticks

Directions:

1. Boil water and rice in a saucepan over high heat. Reduce the heat to medium-low, cover, and cook for 20-25 minutes, or until the rice is soft and the liquid has been absorbed.
2. In a medium glass or ceramic dish, add soy sauce, brown sugar, and cornstarch, stirring until smooth. Stir in the ginger, garlic, and red pepper flakes, then add the chicken and coat well. Cover and refrigerate for at least 15 minutes.
3. Heat 1 tablespoon sesame oil in a wok or big skillet over medium-high heat. Cook and stir in the broccoli, onion, carrots, water chestnuts, and bell pepper for approximately 5 minutes, or until just tender. Transfer vegetables to a plate and set aside.
4. Heat the remaining 1 tablespoon sesame oil in the same wok or skillet over medium-high heat. Cook the chicken until slightly browned, about 2 minutes per side, then toss in the vegetables and leftover marinade. Bring to a boil, then cook and stir until the chicken is no longer pink in the center and the vegetables are cooked, about 5 to 7 minutes. Serve over rice.

Creamy Chicken Pot Pie

Prep: 25 minutes Total: 1 hour and 5 minutes.
Servings:6

Ingredients:

Crust:

- 1 box (14.1 oz) refrigerated Pillsbury Pie Crusts (2 counts), softened as instructed on the box.

Filling:

- 1/3 cup butter or margarine.
- 1/3 cup chopped onion, 1/3 cup all-purpose flour.
- To prepare, combine 1/2 teaspoon salt, 1/4 teaspoon pepper, and 3/4 cup from a 32-ounce carton. Progresso™ Classic Chicken Broth.
- 1/2 cup milk.
- 2 1/2 cup shredded cooked chicken or turkey.
- 2 cups frozen mixed vegetables, thawed

Directions:

1. Preheat oven to 425°F. In a 9-inch glass pie pan, prepare pie crusts according to the directions on the box for Two-Crust Pie.
2. In a 2-quart saucepan, melt the butter over medium heat. Add the onion and simmer for 2 minutes, stirring regularly, until tender. Stir in the flour, salt, and pepper until thoroughly combined. Gradually add the broth and milk, stirring until bubbling and thickened.

3. Stir in the chicken and mixed vegetables. Remove from heat. Spoon the chicken mixture into the crust-lined pan. Top with the second crust, then seal the edge and flute. Cut many slits in the top crust.

4. Bake for 30-40 minutes, or until the crust is golden brown. To prevent excessive browning, wrap the crust border with sheets of foil in the final 15 to 20 minutes of baking. Let stand for 5 minutes before serving.

Mashed Potatoes & Grilled Chicken

Time: one hour.
Serves: 5

Ingredients:

- 6 potatoes.
- 1 teaspoon dried parsley.
- One teaspoon of aromat.
- 2 tablespoons rama.
- 1/2 cup milk.
- 2 kilogram of chicken parts.
- One teaspoon of chicken spice.
- Add 1 teaspoon of paprika.
- Use 1/2 cup beef marinade.

Direction:

1. Peel potatoes and boil in a pot till soft, then add aromat,rama, and milk mix, sprinkle with parsley and mash.

2. Defrost the chicken, then marinade it in a bowl with spices for thirty minutes. Preheat the oven and lightly grease the oven pan with oil before grilling the chicken.
3. Served with cooked beets and chutney.

Meatloaf with Roasted Vegetables

Preparation: 20 minutes.
Inactive: 10 minutes.
Cook: 1 hour and 5 minutes.
Total: 1 hour and 35 minutes.
Servings:6

Ingredients:

- 3 tablespoons olive oil.
- To prepare, coarsely dice one large zucchini and one red bell pepper.
- 1 yellow pepper, coarsely diced
- 5 cloves garlic, crushed into a pulp with coarse salt.
- 1/2 teaspoon of red pepper flakes, split
- salt, and freshly ground black pepper.
- two big eggs, lightly beaten
- 1 tablespoon coarsely chopped fresh thyme leaves.
- 1/4 cup chopped fresh parsley leaves, with more for garnish.
- 1/2 pound of ground pork.
- 1/2-pound ground veal.
- 1 pound of ground beef chuck.
- 1 cup panko (Japanese breadcrumbs)
- 1/2 cup of freshly grated Romano or Parmesan.

- One cup of ketchup, split
- 1/4 cup + 2 teaspoons balsamic vinegar.

Directions:

1. Preheat oven to 425 degrees Fahrenheit.
2. Heat oil in a big saute pan over high heat. Cook the zucchini, peppers, garlic paste, 1/4 teaspoon red pepper flakes, and salt & pepper to taste for 5 minutes, or until almost mushy. Set aside for cooling.
3. Combine eggs and herbs in a large bowl. Combine the meat, bread crumbs, cheese, 1/2 cup ketchup, 2 teaspoons balsamic vinegar, and cooled veggies; stir until just mixed.
4. Place the meatloaf on a baking sheet covered with parchment paper. In a separate bowl, whisk together the remaining ketchup, balsamic vinegar, and red pepper flakes. Brush the mixture over the whole loaf. Bake the meatloaf for 1–1 1/4 hours. Remove from the oven and allow to stand for 10 minutes before slicing.

Tuna Casserole

Prep Time: 10 minutes
Cook time: 20 minutes.
Total Time: 30 minutes.
Servings:6

Ingredients:

- 1 (12 oz.) box egg noodles
- Two (10.5-ounce) cans of condensed cream of mushroom soup

- Divide 2 cups of shredded Cheddar cheese and 2 drained (5-ounce) cans of tuna.
- 1 cup of frozen green peas.
- $\frac{1}{2}$ (4.5 ounce) can of sliced mushrooms
- $\frac{1}{4}$ cup chopped onions
- 1 cup of crumbled potato chips.

Directions:

1. Gather all the ingredients.
2. Bring a big saucepan of lightly salted water to a quick boil. Boil the egg noodles for 7 to 9 minutes, or until soft yet firm to the biting. Drain.
3. Preheat oven to 425 degrees Fahrenheit (220 degrees Celsius).
4. Combine noodles, condensed soup, 1 cup cheese, tuna, peas, mushrooms, and onion in a large bowl until well blended.
5. Transfer the mixture to a 9-by-13-inch baking dish.
6. Top with crumbled potato chips and the remaining 1 cup cheese.
7. Bake in the preheated oven for 15 to 20 minutes, or until the cheese is bubbling.
8. Serve hot, and enjoy!

Pasta Primavera

Preparation time: 20 minutes
Cook time: 15 minutes.
Total time: 35 minutes.
Servings:8

Ingredients:

- 16 ounces penne pasta
- 1 tablespoon of olive oil.
- 8 ounces asparagus, cut into 1 $\frac{1}{2}$-inch pieces.
- 1 yellow bell pepper, sliced into 1 $\frac{1}{2}$ inch pieces.
- 2 cups tiny broccoli florets.
- 1 small zucchini, chopped.
- Add salt and black pepper to taste.
- 2 tablespoons unsalted butter.
- 1 shallot, minced
- 4 garlic cloves, minced
- Zest from 1 lemon
- Dash of crushed red pepper flakes
- 1 cup veggie broth, 1/2 cup heavy cream.
- Three tablespoons of lemon juice, divided
- 1 cup frozen peas.
- 1/2 cup shredded Parmesan cheese.
- 1 $\frac{1}{2}$ cups halved grape tomatoes and $\frac{1}{4}$ cup minced basil.
- 2 tablespoons of Italian parsley, for garnish.
- Extra Parmesan cheese for garnish.
- Crushed red pepper flakes for garnish.

Directions:

1. Heat a big saucepan of water to a boil. Add salt and pasta to the boiling water. Cook for 11 minutes, stirring periodically. Drain well. Pour the spaghetti back into the pot.
2. In a large skillet, heat olive oil over medium-high heat. Combine the asparagus, peppers, and broccoli. Sauté for 2–3 minutes, stirring periodically. Add the zucchini and sauté for 1 to 2 minutes, or until soft but crisp. Season the vegetables with salt and pepper to taste. Move the vegetables to a big plate or bowl.
3. Return the skillet to the stove. Melt the butter over a medium heat. Cook the shallot and garlic for 2 minutes. Mix in the lemon zest and veggie broth. Simmer for 4 to 5 minutes, or until the broth has been reduced by 50%. Mix in the heavy cream and 2 tablespoons of lemon juice.
4. Stir in the peas with the spaghetti. Stir in the cooked vegetables. Pour the lemon cream sauce over the pasta and vegetables, stirring until thoroughly mixed. Mix in the Parmesan cheese and the remaining tablespoon of fresh lemon juice. Gently mix in the tomatoes and basil. Season with salt and black pepper to taste.
5. Transfer the pasta primavera to a large serving bowl or platter. Garnish with parsley, additional Parmesan, and crushed red pepper flakes. Serve warm.

Beef Stew

Prep time: 15 minutes.
Total time: 1 hour, 40 minutes.
Servings:8

Ingredients:

- 1 tablespoon (or more) of vegetable oil.
- 2 pound. beef chuck stew meat cut into 1-inch chunks
- To prepare, chop one medium yellow onion and peel and cut two carrots into rounds.
- 2 celery stalks, diced with kosher salt.
- Freshly ground black pepper.
- 3 garlic cloves, finely chopped
- 1/4 cup tomato paste.
- 6 cups low-sodium beef broth.
- 1 cup red wine.
- 1 tablespoon Worcestershire sauce.
- Two fresh thyme sprigs.
- Two bay leaves.
- 1 pound baby potatoes, halved.
- 1 cup frozen peas.
- 1/4 cup chopped fresh parsley.

Directions:

1. Heat oil in a large Dutch oven or heavy pot over medium heat. Add the beef and cook, rotating regularly, until it is charred on all sides, about 10 minutes. Transfer the beef to a dish.
2. Coat the bottom of the pot with oil if necessary and heat on medium-high. Cook the onion, carrots, and celery, turning

occasionally, until softened, about 7 minutes. Season with salt and pepper. Cook, stirring, until the garlic is aromatic and the tomato paste darkens about 2 minutes. Return beef to the pot. Combine the broth, wine, Worcestershire, thyme, and bay leaves. Bring to a boil, then decrease heat to medium-low and simmer; season with salt and pepper. Cover and cook, stirring occasionally, until the beef is cooked, about 30 to 45 minutes.

3. Cover and boil potatoes until cooked, approximately 15 minutes.
4. Remove bay leaves and thyme. Stir in the peas and cook for approximately 2 minutes, stirring occasionally, until warmed through. Season with salt and pepper.
5. Divide stew among bowls. Top with parsley.

Tofu Scramble with Vegetables

Prep:10minutes
Cook:15minutes
Total:30minutes
Servings: 2-4 servings

Ingredients:

- Two tablespoons of cooking oil.
- 1 small red bell pepper, chopped
- 1/2 yellow onion, chopped
- 1 garlic clove, minced
- One (16-ounce) package of firm tofu.
- Two cups of baby spinach (optional)
- 1 cup polenta (optional).

- Two tablespoons of vegan margarine.
- One spoonful of turmeric.
- 1 tablespoon nutritional yeast (optional).
- One teaspoon of oregano.
- Add salt and pepper to taste.

Directions:

1. In a large frying pan, sauté the bell pepper, onions, and garlic in the majority of the oil for a few minutes.
2. Crumble the tofu into the pan with your fingers and swirl to combine.
3. If you're using polenta (it makes it incredibly wet, like scrambled eggs, but we only use this recipe when we have extra polenta), toss it in and stir.
4. Next, add the spinach and vegan margarine, melt it, and toss to coat the tofu crumbles. Add the turmeric and nutritional yeast (optional) and stir once more.
5. Add most of your vegetables. If you're using longer-cooking vegetables like broccoli, carrots, or potatoes, cook them for about 10 minutes before adding fast-cooking veggies like mushrooms, kale, spinach, and tomatoes. You should simmer the entire mixture for around 15 minutes.
6. Turn off the heat and let aside for a few minutes before serving.

Part III: High-Fiber Diet

After you've recovered from a Diverticulitis attack, your doctor will urge you to increase your fiber intake. Consuming more fiber, or taking fiber supplements, can help prevent future attacks.

This is because fiber softens feces and prevents constipation. Avoiding constipation helps to reduce intestinal pressure, which may avoid future Diverticulitis flare-ups.

However, when it comes to eating extra fiber, start cautiously. Begin by consuming 5–15 grams of fiber per day. Start with a small amount of fiber and gradually increase your regular intake. If you are experiencing bloating or gas, limit your fiber intake for a few days.

As you add additional fiber, keep track of your hydration intake. Fibers require water to function correctly. If you don't drink enough water, your stools can become overly stiff and difficult to pass.

The following high-fiber diets are indicated to treat Diverticulitis:

a)Beans and legumes.

b)   Bran, whole wheat bread, oatmeal, and other whole grain cereals

c)Brown Rice, Quinoa, and Barley

d)   Fruits including strawberries, apples, pears, kiwis, and oranges

e)   vegetables including broccoli, cauliflower, carrots, and dark leafy greens (kale, collard greens, Swiss chard, and spinach).

f)Whole wheat pasta.

g)Popcorn

h)   Nuts and Seeds

Breakfast Recipes

Chia Pudding with Fruit and Nuts

Ingredients:

- 1 cup almond milk
- 1 cup coconut milk
- 1 cup Greek yogurt.
- ·1 tablespoon honey
- 1 teaspoon vanilla
- $\frac{3}{4}$ cup chia seeds
- chopped pears
- apples
- almonds
- pomegranate seeds for garnish

Directions:

1. In a large bowl, combine almond milk, coconut milk, yogurt, honey, and vanilla.
2. Combine and fold in chia seeds. Refrigerate for 4 to 6 hours in an airtight container.
3. Garnish with fruit and nuts and serve cool.

Overnight oatmeal with apples and walnuts

Ingredients:

- $\frac{1}{2}$ cup rolled oats
- $\frac{1}{2}$ cup unsweetened vanilla soy milk
- 1 tablespoon chia seeds

- $\frac{1}{2}$ cup chopped apples
- 1 teaspoon maple syrup
- $\frac{1}{4}$ teaspoon apple pie spice
- $\frac{1}{4}$ cup apple cider or apple juice
- 1 teaspoon lemon juice
- A pinch of salt.

Directions:

1. To make overnight oats, combine soy milk, chia seeds, maple syrup, salt, and apple pie spice in a mason jar. Stir vigorously to prevent the chia seeds from sticking together.
2. Refrigerate overnight (12-24 hours).
3. To serve, add chopped apples, crumbled walnuts, or your favorite oatmeal toppings.

High Fiber Smoothie Bowl

Ingredients:

- 1 Fiber One Lemon Drizzle Square (90 calories) broken into small pieces.
- One medium banana.
- 150g strawberries (stems removed), 70g raspberries, 60g blackberries, and 200ml apple juice.
- Combine 1 tablespoon mixed seeds (e.g. sunflower and pumpkin seeds) with 10g halved hazelnuts.

Directions:

1. Combine the banana, 100g strawberries, 50g raspberries, and
   25g blackberries in a blender with apple juice. Whizz until
   smooth. Pour into a serving bowl.
2. Slice any remaining strawberries. Place strawberry slices, the
   remaining raspberries and blackberries, and lemon square
   pieces in rows on top of the smoothie. Sprinkle with mixed
   seeds and hazelnuts. Serve right away.

Banana Flaxseed Muffins

Prep:10minutes
Cook:25minutes
Total:35minutes
Servings:6

Ingredients:

- 3/4 cup mashed ripe bananas
- 1 large egg
- 2 Tbsp brown sugar
- 1/2 tsp vanilla
- 2 Tbsp olive oil
- 1 cup all-purpose flour
- 1 tsp baking powder
- 1/4 cup ground flaxseed
- 1/4 cup chopped walnuts (optional)

Direction:

1. Preheat oven to 425°F. In a medium bowl, combine the mashed
   banana, egg, brown sugar, vanilla, and olive oil.

2. In a separate medium bowl, combine flour, baking powder, salt, flaxseed, and walnuts.
3. Combine wet and dry ingredients, stirring until no flour remains on the bottom of the bowl. Avoid over-stirring the batter.
4. Line six muffin tray wells with paper liners. Divide batter evenly between them. It should fill the wells close to the top.
5. Bake the muffins at 425°F for five minutes, then decrease to 350°F without opening the oven door and continue baking for 20 minutes.
6. Once baked, remove the muffins from the tray to cool. Enjoy the muffins right away, or let them cool completely before storing them in an airtight container in the fridge.

Probiotic-rich foods like yogurt, kefir, and fermented vegetables can help to maintain a healthy balance of gut flora and improve digestive health.

Lunch Recipes

Quinoa Salad with Grilled Chicken

Preparation time: 10 minutes.
Cook time: 30 minutes.
Total time is 40 minutes.
servings:8.

Ingredients:

- Four tablespoons of olive oil, divided
- one cup of raw quinoa (I used rainbow quinoa)
- two and a half teaspoons of salt, divided
- additional salt to taste
- two cups of chicken or vegetable broth
- one pound of boneless chicken breasts or thighs
- one and a half teaspoons of black pepper
- two ears of corn on the cob
- one red bell pepper, chopped
- one and a half cups of toasted pine nuts
- one small bunch of chopped basil
- and one small bunch of chopped basil

Directions:

1. Warm 1 tablespoon olive oil in a small saucepan over medium heat. Stir in the quinoa and 1 teaspoon salt until evenly incorporated. Bring the chicken or vegetable stock to a boil.
2. Turn the heat down to low and cover. Cook for 15 minutes, then remove from heat and cover for a further 5 minutes. Fluff with a fork.
3. Season chicken breasts with 1 teaspoon salt and pepper. Cook on a medium-high grill until the internal temperature reaches

160°F, which should take about 12-17 minutes depending on the size of the chicken breasts. Remove from the grill and let cool slightly. Chop into ½-inch pieces.

4. Brush the corn cobs with 1 tablespoon olive oil and season with salt and pepper while cooking the chicken.
5. Place on the grill and cook for 5-7 minutes, flipping occasionally. Remove from the grill and use a knife to separate the corn kernels from the cob.
6. In a large bowl, combine quinoa, chicken, corn, red pepper, pine nuts, half of the feta cheese, and half of the basil. Garnish with the remaining cheese and basil. Serve either warm or cold.

Lentil Soup with Whole-Grain Bread

Prep time: 15 minutes.
Cook time: 45 minutes.
Serves:4

Ingredients:

- 1 cup (dry) lentils.
- 2 tablespoons olive oil.
- 1 medium chopped onion, 2 peeled and diced. Carrots
- Two stalks, diced Celery, and minced garlic (3 cloves)
- Two tablespoons. Tomato paste
- One can (14.5 ounces). Diced tomatoes.
- 4 cups Vegetable broth (1 teaspoon) Ground cumin (1/2 teaspoon) ground coriander, 1 bay leaf.
- Salt to taste.

- Add black pepper to taste.
- Two tablespoons. Use fresh lemon juice for garnish. Fresh parsley or cilantro.

For serving:

- Whole grain bread. Two slices for each person.
- Optional additives for increased flavor or nutrition:
- Red pepper flakes: add a pinch for heat.
- For extra nutrients, add a handful of spinach or kale toward the end.
- Grated Parmesan cheese for garnish.

Directions:

1. Rinse the lentils in cold water. Drain them and set aside.
2. In a big pot or Dutch oven, heat olive oil over medium heat. When the oil is hot, add the chopped onions, carrots, and celery. Cook for 5–7 minutes, or until the vegetables begin to soften.
3. Cook the minced garlic for another minute until fragrant.
4. Stir in tomato paste and simmer for another 2 minutes.
5. Combine chopped tomatoes, vegetable broth, lentils, ground cumin, ground coriander, bay leaf, salt, and black pepper in the pot. Heat everything to a boil.
6. Once boiling, reduce heat to medium and simmer for 30-40 minutes until lentils are cooked.

7. While simmering, taste and adjust seasonings as needed. If you're using red pepper flakes, spinach, or kale, add them in the final 5 minutes of cooking.
8. Once the lentils are cooked and soft, remove them from the fire. Take out and discard the bay leaf. Stir in the fresh lemon juice.
9. For a smoother texture, use an immersion blender to partially mix the soup while keeping some chunks for texture.
10.   Garnish the soup with fresh parsley or cilantro and optional grated Parmesan cheese.

Vegetable Wrap With Hummus and Sprouts

Ingredients:

- 1 flavored wrap or tortilla (I used spinach)
- ⅓ cup hummus
- 2 sliced cucumbers (lengthwise)
- Handful of fresh spinach leaves
- Slicing tomato (depending on size)
- ¼ avocado, fresh alfalfa or broccoli sprouts, and fresh microgreens.
- Optional: add basil leaves.

Directions:

1. Spread the hummus on the bottom ⅓ of the wrap, leaving about ½ inch from the bottom edge and spreading out to the sides.
2. Layer cucumber, spinach, tomato, avocado, sprouts, microgreens, and basil.
3. Fold the wrap tightly like a burrito, tucking in all the veggies with the initial roll and rolling hard till the finish. Cut in half and enjoy.

Chicken Stir-Fry with Brown Rice and Broccoli

Preparation: 10 minutes.
Cook: 20 minutes.
Servings: Two.

Ingredients:

- 200g broccoli florets (about 6), halved
- 1 chicken breast (approx 180g), diced
- 15g ginger, cut into shreds
- 2 garlic cloves, cut into shreds
- 1 red onion, sliced
- 1 roasted red pepper, cut into cubes
- 2 tsp olive oil
- 1 tsp mild chili powder
- 1 tbsp reduced-salt soy sauce
- 1 tbsp honey
- 250g cooked brown rice

Directions:

1. Put the kettle on to boil, then place the broccoli in a medium pan ready to cook. Pour the water over the broccoli and boil for 4 minutes.

2. Heat the olive oil in a nonstick wok and stir-fry
   the ginger, garlic, and onion for 2 minutes before
   adding the mild chili powder and stirring briefly.
3. Stir in the chicken and cook for an additional two
   minutes. Drain the broccoli and save the water.
4. Cook the broccoli in the wok with the soy sauce,
   honey, red pepper, and 4 tablespoons of broccoli
   water until heated through. Meanwhile, cook the
   rice according to package instructions and serve
   with the stir-fry.

Dinner Recipes

Stuffed Sweet Potatoes with Black Beans

Total time: 1 hour and 10 minutes.
Serves: 4

Ingredients:

- 4 medium-large sweet potatoes
- 1/2 cup cashew cream sauce (optional sour cream or plain Greek yogurt if not vegan)
- 1 teaspoon lime juice
- 1/2 teaspoon ground black pepper
- 1/2 medium red onion, finely chopped (approximately 1 cup)
- 1 1/2 teaspoons oil (I used olive oil)
- 1/4 teaspoon garlic powder.
- 1/4 teaspoon onion powder
- 1/4 teaspoon cumin
- 1/4 teaspoon chili powder
- 1/2 teaspoon sea salt
- 1 15oz can of black beans (drained and washed).

For Serving:

- Chop 1/2 avocado.
- Chop a handful of Cilantro.

Directions:

1. Preheat the oven to 350 degrees F.
2. Place the sweet potatoes on a lightly greased baking tray and bake for 55-65 minutes, or until a fork easily pierces the flesh.

3. To make the cream sauce, combine cashew cream sauce, lime juice, and black pepper. Set aside.
4. Heat oil in a skillet over medium heat and add onion after about 10 minutes of cooking sweet potatoes. Saute the onions for 5 minutes, or until they become translucent. Add the spices, mix, and simmer for another 3 minutes.
5. Toss the black beans in the skillet. Continue cooking, stirring regularly, until the black beans are completely cooked through. Approximately 5 minutes. Turn off the heat and set aside.
6. After baking, allow the sweet potatoes to cool somewhat. When the sweet potatoes have cooled, split them open and shred the flesh from the skin until the inside is mashed and simple to scoop out.
7. Evenly distribute the black bean mixture, avocado, cilantro, and cashew crema sauce over the four sweet potatoes.
8. Serve immediately and enjoy!

Lentil Bolognese

Prep Time: 10 minutes
Cook Time: 45 minutes.
Total Time: 55 minutes

Ingredients:

- 1 cup lentils
- 3 cups water
- 2 tablespoons olive oil
- 1 chopped onion

- 3 cloves garlic minced
- 2 grated carrots
- 2 celery stalks chopped
- 28 oz crushed tomatoes
- $\frac{1}{2}$ teaspoon paprika
- 1 tablespoon apple cider vinegar
- 1 teaspoon vegan worcheshire sauce (optional but tasty)
- Salt and pepper to taste
- 12 ounces pasta

Toppings:

- Fresh parsley

Directions:

1. In a pot, combine 1 cup of lentils with 3 cups water. Cook until the lentils are cooked (approximately 15-20 minutes). Drain the the lentils and discard any remaining water in the pot.
2. In a big pan/pot, combine oil, onion, and garlic and cook for 5 minutes until transparent.
3. Combine carrots, celery, tomatoes, paprika, apple cider vinegar, vegan worcheshire sauce, salt, and pepper. Cook for 10 minutes.
4. Cook pasta according to package directions while the vegetables are cooking.
5. Cook for 5 minutes more, or until lentils and carrots are cooked.

6. Place spaghetti in dishes, and top with lentil bolognese, parsley.

Roasted Vegetable Couscous Bowl

Prep Time: 20 minutes
Total time: 1 hour, servings: 4

Ingredients:

- Rinse and drain 1 can (14 ounces) of chickpeas
- Trim and cut 1 head of cauliflower (1 $\frac{1}{2}$ pounds) into quarters
- Peel and cut 8 ounces (approximately 4 carrots) into 1-inch pieces.
- $\frac{1}{4}$ cup extra virgin olive oil, with more for drizzling
- $\frac{1}{4}$ teaspoon ras el hanout (a Moroccan spice blend) or curry powder.
- Halved lemon
- Kosher salt and freshly ground pepper
- 10 oz couscous
- 4 oz crumbled feta (1 cup)
- $\frac{1}{4}$ cup coarsely chopped cilantro

Directions:

1. Preheat oven to 475 degrees. Place a rimmed baking sheet on the center rack. Toss the chickpeas, cauliflower, and carrots with oil and ras el hanout.
2. Transfer to a heated baking sheet with the lemon halves, cut sides up; season with salt and pepper. Roast for 30 minutes,

until browned and mostly tender. Remove from the oven and reserve the lemon.

3. Reduce heat to 350 degrees. On a baking sheet, combine couscous, 2 cups boiling water, and 1 teaspoon salt; stir. Wearing oven mitts, cover the sheet with parchment-lined foil and crimp the edges securely; carefully return to the oven.

4. Cook for ten minutes, or until the liquid has been absorbed. Remove from the oven and cool for 5 minutes, covered. Remove the foil, squeeze the reserved lemon over the couscous, and fluff with a fork. Finish with feta, cilantro, and a drizzle of oil; serve.

Lentil Shepherd's Pie

Preparation time: than 20 minutes
Cooking time: 30 minutes to one hour.
Serves: 4

Ingredients:

For the champ topping:

- Peel and cut 3 floury potatoes, such as King Edward or Maris Piper
- . Add frozen peas and a knob of butter.
- Roughly slice 2 spring onions.
- Add 25ml/1fl oz milk.
- Break up 75g/3oz mature cheddar into chunks.
- Sprinkle with smoky paprika.

For the lentil mix:

- 1 tbsp olive oil
- $\frac{1}{2}$ red onion, roughly chopped
- 1 garlic clove, chopped
- 2 small carrots, peeled and sliced into tiny pieces
- 1 celery stalk, trimmed and chopped into small pieces
- 400g/14oz canned plum tomatoes
- Worcestershire sauce (optional)
- A few drops of Tabasco
- smoked paprika
- 1 fresh bay leaf
- 85ml/3fl oz red wine.
- 100ml (3$\frac{1}{2}$fl oz) vegetable stock
- 1 sprig of fresh rosemary
- Balsamic vinegar
- Small handful of chopped fresh flat-leaf parsley
- 400g/14oz canned Puy lentils
- Sea salt and freshly ground black pepper

Directions:

1. Preheat oven to 200C (400F/Gas). 6. For the champ topping, heat a pan of salted water, add the potatoes, and bring to a gentle boil before simmering for 15-20 minutes, or until nearly cooked through. When the potatoes for the champ topping are about done, add the frozen peas and simmer for a few minutes longer, or until soft. Drain and set aside.

2. In a large frying pan, heat olive oil over medium heat. Cook onion, garlic, carrots, and celery for 5-10 minutes until softened.

3. Season to taste with salt and freshly ground black pepper, then add the remaining lentil mixture components (except lentils). Bring to a boil, then reduce heat and simmer for 10 minutes, or until the veggies are soft and the sauce is reduced. Stir the lentils into the tomato sauce.

4. In a small skillet, melt butter over low heat and gently cook spring onions until tender. Add the milk and heat through.

5. Mash potatoes and peas roughly. Add the warm milk mixture to the potatoes and mash until smooth but still lumpy.

6. Transfer the lentil mixture to a medium pie dish and top with champ. Sprinkle with the cheese and smoked paprika. Place the pie on a baking sheet and bake for 25-30 minutes, or until the potatoes are golden brown.

Conclusion:
when can I resume my normal diet?

Once your Diverticulitis symptoms have subsided, you can gradually and mindfully introduce other healthy foods back into your diet. However, it may take a week or more before you can resume your regular eating habits. Your healthcare practitioner will advise you on when and how to resume a normal diet.

Thank You

I just wanted to take a moment to say a huge thank you for choosing to read this book. I hope you enjoyed it and found it helpful! As authors, we truly value reviews on Amazon, and your positive feedback would mean the world to us. By leaving a review, you'll not only help us reach more readers but also assist others in discovering the true value of this book.

I know your time is precious, so I genuinely appreciate your willingness to share your thoughts with us. Thank you in advance for considering leaving a kind review. Your support is incredibly important to us!

Warmest regards,

8-Week Meal Planner

WEEK _______________________

MONTH _______________________

MONDAY
BREAKFAST:

LUNCH:

DINNER:

SNACK:

TUESDAY
BREAKFAST:

LUNCH:

DINNER:

SNACK:

WEDNESDAY
BREAKFAST:

LUNCH:

DINNER:

SNACK:

THURSDAY
BREAKFAST:

LUNCH:

DINNER:

SNACK:

FRIDAY
BREAKFAST:

LUNCH:

DINNER:

SNACK:

SATURDAY
BREAKFAST:

LUNCH:

DINNER:

SNACK:

SUNDAY
BREAKFAST:

LUNCH:

DINNER:

SNACK:

NOTES

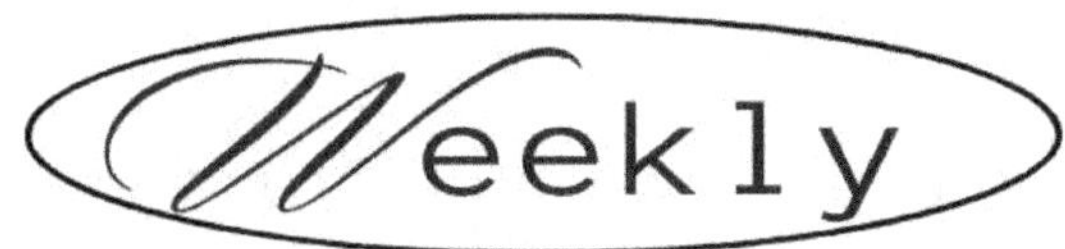 Weekly MEAL PLANNER

WEEK _______________________ **MONTH** _______________________

MONDAY
BREAKFAST:

LUNCH:

DINNER:

SNACK:

TUESDAY
BREAKFAST:

LUNCH:

DINNER:

SNACK:

WEDNESDAY
BREAKFAST:

LUNCH:

DINNER:

SNACK:

THURSDAY
BREAKFAST:

LUNCH:

DINNER:

SNACK:

FRIDAY
BREAKFAST:

LUNCH:

DINNER:

SNACK:

SATURDAY
BREAKFAST:

LUNCH:

DINNER:

SNACK:

SUNDAY
BREAKFAST:

LUNCH:

DINNER:

SNACK:

NOTES

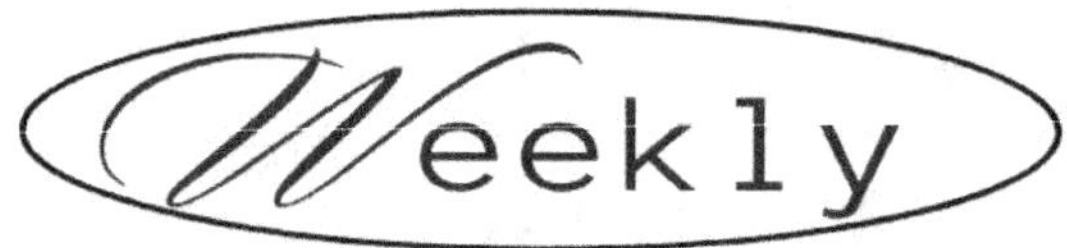

MEAL PLANNER

WEEK _______________________

MONTH _______________________

MONDAY
BREAKFAST:

LUNCH:

DINNER:

SNACK:

TUESDAY
BREAKFAST:

LUNCH:

DINNER:

SNACK:

WEDNESDAY
BREAKFAST:

LUNCH:

DINNER:

SNACK:

THURSDAY
BREAKFAST:

LUNCH:

DINNER:

SNACK:

FRIDAY
BREAKFAST:

LUNCH:

DINNER:

SNACK:

SATURDAY
BREAKFAST:

LUNCH:

DINNER:

SNACK:

SUNDAY
BREAKFAST:

LUNCH:

DINNER:

SNACK:

NOTES

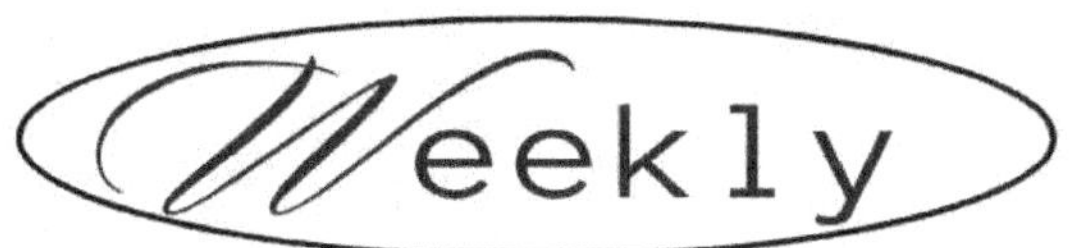

MEAL PLANNER

WEEK ___________________   **MONTH** ___________________

MONDAY
BREAKFAST:

LUNCH:

DINNER:

SNACK:

TUESDAY
BREAKFAST:

LUNCH:

DINNER:

SNACK:

WEDNESDAY
BREAKFAST:

LUNCH:

DINNER:

SNACK:

THURSDAY
BREAKFAST:

LUNCH:

DINNER:

SNACK:

FRIDAY
BREAKFAST:

LUNCH:

DINNER:

SNACK:

SATURDAY
BREAKFAST:

LUNCH:

DINNER:

SNACK:

SUNDAY
BREAKFAST:

LUNCH:

DINNER:

SNACK:

NOTES

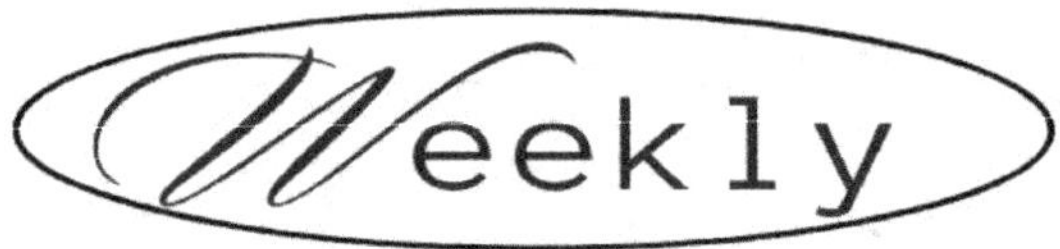

MEAL PLANNER

WEEK _______________________ MONTH _______________________

MONDAY
BREAKFAST:

LUNCH:

DINNER:

SNACK:

TUESDAY
BREAKFAST:

LUNCH:

DINNER:

SNACK:

WEDNESDAY
BREAKFAST:

LUNCH:

DINNER:

SNACK:

THURSDAY
BREAKFAST:

LUNCH:

DINNER:

SNACK:

FRIDAY
BREAKFAST:

LUNCH:

DINNER:

SNACK:

SATURDAY
BREAKFAST:

LUNCH:

DINNER:

SNACK:

SUNDAY
BREAKFAST:

LUNCH:

DINNER:

SNACK:

NOTES

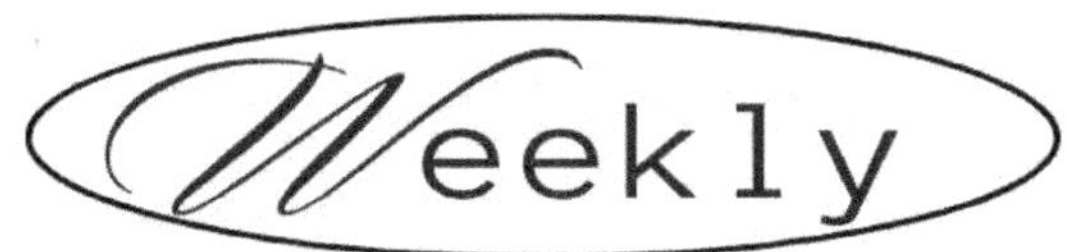

MEAL PLANNER

WEEK _________________________   **MONTH** _________________________

MONDAY
BREAKFAST:

LUNCH:

DINNER:

SNACK:

TUESDAY
BREAKFAST:

LUNCH:

DINNER:

SNACK:

WEDNESDAY
BREAKFAST:

LUNCH:

DINNER:

SNACK:

THURSDAY
BREAKFAST:

LUNCH:

DINNER:

SNACK:

FRIDAY
BREAKFAST:

LUNCH:

DINNER:

SNACK:

SATURDAY
BREAKFAST:

LUNCH:

DINNER:

SNACK:

SUNDAY
BREAKFAST:

LUNCH:

DINNER:

SNACK:

NOTES

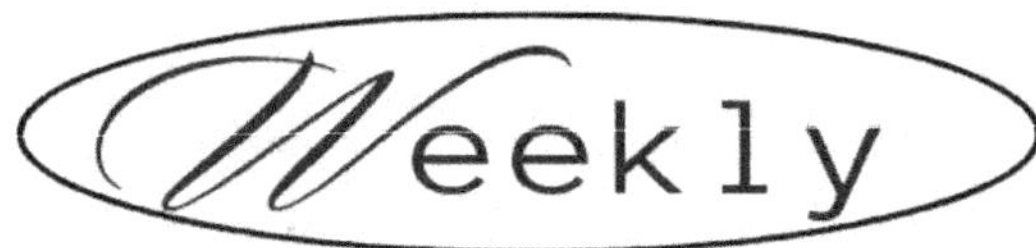

MEAL PLANNER

WEEK ___________________________   **MONTH** ___________________________

MONDAY
BREAKFAST:

LUNCH:

DINNER:

SNACK:

TUESDAY
BREAKFAST:

LUNCH:

DINNER:

SNACK:

WEDNESDAY
BREAKFAST:

LUNCH:

DINNER:

SNACK:

THURSDAY
BREAKFAST:

LUNCH:

DINNER:

SNACK:

FRIDAY
BREAKFAST:

LUNCH:

DINNER:

SNACK:

SATURDAY
BREAKFAST:

LUNCH:

DINNER:

SNACK:

SUNDAY
BREAKFAST:

LUNCH:

DINNER:

SNACK:

NOTES

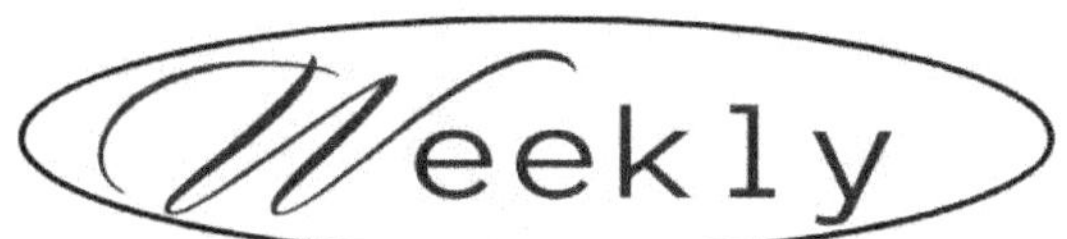

MEAL PLANNER

WEEK _______________________

MONTH _______________________

MONDAY
BREAKFAST:

LUNCH:

DINNER:

SNACK:

TUESDAY
BREAKFAST:

LUNCH:

DINNER:

SNACK:

WEDNESDAY
BREAKFAST:

LUNCH:

DINNER:

SNACK:

THURSDAY
BREAKFAST:

LUNCH:

DINNER:

SNACK:

FRIDAY
BREAKFAST:

LUNCH:

DINNER:

SNACK:

SATURDAY
BREAKFAST:

LUNCH:

DINNER:

SNACK:

SUNDAY
BREAKFAST:

LUNCH:

DINNER:

SNACK:

NOTES

If you're not sure which foods to include or avoid in your diverticulitis diet, it's always a good idea to speak with a certified dietitian or healthcare expert for tailored advice.

Recipe Index